Scientific Faith

How to Bridge the Gap Between God and Science

TS Taylor

All for the Glory of God

Table of Contents

How to Use This Guide

Introduction

You may find this study guide to be somewhat different from other study guides in that its focus is on the intersection of science and the Christian faith. The studies within this book are not meant to be exhaustive, but as a start to a new way of thinking about some perplexing issues.

The main purpose is to present a classic Christian view in light of modern society's view. You might learn some new ideas and some new language that you can use to communicate with your friends and neighbors about who God is and what Jesus has done for us all.

As You Read

Feel free to read at your own pace. This is not intended to be an exhaustive study or have deep and complex scientific equations. Therefore, you may want to do some independent research on your own with issues that strike you deeply.

Pray that the Holy Spirit would help the mediations of your heart to be acceptable in God's sight (Psalm 19:14).

Enjoy the questions. They are meant to be open-ended. As such, some of the questions may bring multiple perspectives. If one resonates with you, feel free to ask other deeper questions along the same path.

Personal Study or Small Group?

This book can be used for either personal study or with a small group. If you use it with a small group, think about how best to use your time together.

Pray together. Ask God to open your hearts and minds so that the time together would honor Him and deepen the faith of all involved.

Summarize and discuss. Have one or two people in the group summarize the Session for this meeting. Ask everyone what they particularly liked (or disliked) about this writing and what for them was encouraging or challenging.

Questions. Talk through the discussion questions at the end of each Session. Listen carefully to what others in the group say, as they may be touching on deeper issues. Feel free to allow some questions to take you into a deeper discussion. Also, feel free to table a deeper scientific discussion until another time, to allow those interested to do some more research. Then discuss this at a later time.

Application. How can you use any of these discussions to have deeper conversations about faith with your friends and neighbors? If you have a specific friend in mind, ask others to pray along with you as you seek to discuss your faith more deeply with them.

Rejoice. Above all, rejoice in the richness and majesty of God and how He reveals Himself in His creation.

For more information join us at *https://www.tstaylorbooks.com/*.

An Introduction: A Literal Bible and Exhaustive Knowledge?

The First Step: Should We Take the Bible Literally?

When it comes to the study of faith and science, one of the first questions that often comes to mind is, "Do you take the Bible literally?" Oddly enough, the correct answer to this question is, "Of course, yes." This is because what the question is asking is, "Do you take the Bible in the manner in which it was written?" Of course, what other way is there to read any work of literature?

Many people do not realize that the Bible is written in many different literary genres. There is poetry, wisdom literature, didactic literature, and of course historical narrative. Sometimes it takes real work to figure out what literary genre is being used, but with just a bit of careful reading, it is fairly easy to discover the truth.

> *¹ The LORD is my shepherd; I shall not want. ² He makes me to lie down in green pastures; He leads me beside the still waters. (Psalm 23:1–2)*

This is a fairly famous Psalm by King David, written thousands of years ago. David is not trying to convey the idea that God is literally a shepherd in Israel, walking around dusty fields with a flock of sheep. He is giving God human attributes in this way to make it easier for us to better understand who God is and what He is like. David is trying to convey the idea that God loves His people and takes care of His people as a shepherd loves and cares for his sheep. Shepherds are very good at balancing the good of the entire flock with the rescue of one lost sheep. This is also very true with our heavenly Father.

> *The proverbs of Solomon: A wise son makes a glad father, But a foolish son is the grief of his mother. (Proverbs 10:1)*

Solomon is giving a pithy couplet to get across the idea of honoring your parents. He compares a wise son to a foolish son. It is meant to be read as a wise saying that is true throughout the ages. This couplet is a typical Hebrew literary technique called

parallelism. The verse above is an antithetic parallelism, comparing two different ideas to make a point.

> *As vinegar to the teeth and smoke to the eyes, so*
> *is the lazy man to those who send him. (Proverbs*
> *10:16)*

This proverb is called a synonymous parallelism, as the two lines convey the same idea but in different ways.

> *13 You shall not murder.*
> *14 You shall not commit adultery.*
> *15 You shall not steal. (Exodus 20:13–15)*

Of course, in the Bible, there is the law, a clear description of right and wrong. It is meant to teach us how to live a good and righteous life.

Moses is declaring the moral law of God. It is meant to be taken as a rule or a measure of how to live. These laws are an important part of all societies, throughout time and throughout the globe.

> *1 Now Moses was tending the flock of Jethro his*
> *father-in-law, the priest of Midian. And he led the*
> *flock to the back of the desert, and came to Horeb,*
> *the mountain of God. 2 And the Angel of the LORD*
> *appeared to him in a flame of fire from the midst*
> *of a bush. So he looked, and behold, the bush was*

burning with fire, but the bush was not consumed.
(Exodus 3:1–2)

This is an example of a historical narrative. It gives the name of a real person and how he is related to others at that time. It gives his occupation and his location. It is meant to set the stage for a real event that takes place in space and time. In this historical narrative, God shows up miraculously. The fact that God shows up miraculously does not negate the truth of the historical narrative.

For you shall go out with joy,
And be led out with peace;
The mountains and the hills
Shall break forth into singing before you,
And all the trees of the field shall clap their
hands. (Isaiah 55:12)

This verse above is clearly Hebrew poetry. This section of Isaiah is expressing the joy of the Creation and what it means to be in a right relationship with God. The image of the mountains singing and the trees clapping their hands is meant to be very dramatic and breathtaking.

So, when reading any part of the Bible, the first step is understanding how the section was written and meant to be read. The next time that you read from the Bible, think about what genre of literature is being used, and then read the passage in that context. We will use this literary tool as we go through this study.

Discussion Questions

1. What children's stories are favorites of yours that teach great moral lessons that you don't take "literally"?

2. Can you think of other descriptions of God, like the shepherd? Why do you suppose the Bible uses these different descriptors?

3. Have you ever experienced the mountains singing and the trees clapping their hands, metaphorically? How would you describe that event? How did it make you feel?

4. How can you apply the five W's—who, what, where, when, and why—to better understand a historical narrative in the Bible? Pick a Biblical story and try it out.

5. What friend can you think of that would be surprised if you told them that the Bible had songs and poems in it? Why would they be surprised?

The Second Step: True Knowledge vs. Exhaustive Knowledge

It has been said that the Bible gives true knowledge but does not give exhaustive knowledge.

Does this strike you as a surprising statement? Does it make sense that the Bible can give true knowledge but not exhaustive knowledge?

Firstly, the Bible is fundamentally a book about God. It is about who He is, what He is like, what He loves, and what He hates. Secondly, it is a book about humans, who we are, what we should be like, what we should love, and what we should hate. The Bible is written in a way to help us see that we need to know who God is before we can really know who we are.

Given this premise, does the Bible tell us everything there is to know about God? Unfortunately, no. God is so much bigger than we are, we cannot ever totally comprehend Him. After all, what does it mean to be all-powerful and omniscient (all-knowing)? As much are we learn and study, we will never learn all that there is to know about God. For example, God describes Himself as being very far beyond our comprehension:

> [8] *"For My thoughts are not your thoughts, Nor are your ways My ways," says the LORD.* [9] *"For as the heavens are higher than the earth, So are My ways higher than your ways, And My thoughts than your thoughts." (Isaiah 55:8–9)*

In its quest to tell us who we are, does the Bible tell us everything that we need to know? Unfortunately, no, the Bible does not give exhaustive knowledge.

For example, in ancient Israel as well as today, a sharp blade was important. It is important to us in the kitchen, to surgeons in the operating room, and to the ancient Israelites in preparing for battle. Accordingly, the Bible talks about the importance of keeping your blade sharp, but it does not tell you how to do that because even the Israelites did not know how to sharpen their farming tools. God did not tell them, and they had not figured it out yet; so, they had to go to their sometimes-enemies, the Philistines, to get their tools sharpened.

> [19] *Now there was no blacksmith to be found throughout all the land of Israel, for the Philistines said, "Lest the Hebrews make swords or spears." [20] But all the Israelites would go down to the Philistines to sharpen each man's plowshare, his mattock, his ax, and his sickle... (1 Samuel 13:19–20)*

Another area of limited knowledge is angels. The Bible talks a great deal about angels. A good example of this is the famous verse where Gabriel comes to Mary with his big announcement.

> [26] *Now in the sixth month the angel Gabriel was sent by God to a city of Galilee named Nazareth,*

^{27} to a virgin betrothed to a man whose name was Joseph, of the house of David. The virgin's name was Mary. ^{28} And having come in, the angel said to her, "Rejoice, highly favored one, the Lord is with you; blessed are you among women!"

^{29} But when she saw him, she was troubled at his saying, and considered what manner of greeting this was. (Luke 1:26–29)

The Bible is pretty clear about some aspects of angels, such as the fact that they exist, they have their own names, and they are frightful in appearance. The Bible tells us what we need to know about angels, but it leaves out an awful lot of interesting facts. Take, for example, the following questions: How tall was Gabriel? Did he have a body like you and me, or did he have some kind of ethereal body? Did he have wings? If so, what did they look like? God tells us what we need to know about angels, and we can learn the rest when we get to heaven.

Not only does the Bible not tell us everything, it also often describes events using phenomenological or descriptive language. For example, what is scientifically wrong with the following passage?

^{3} From the rising of the sun to its going down The LORD's name is to be praised. (Psalm 113:3)

Of course, the sun does not move around the earth so it cannot rise or go down. Copernicus and Galileo convinced us of this idea hundreds of years ago. Yet, surprisingly we still use these same expressions today. Most weather apps today will tell you the exact time that "sunrise" and "sunset" will occur, even though this is scientifically incorrect. Often, we will see phenomenological language in the Bible that is meant to describe the event and it is not meant to give an exhaustive, scientifically correct description. It is a description that works in everyday life.

In the Gospel of Matthew, after Jesus cast out the demons in two demon-possessed men, the multitude that witnessed this act was in awe and shock. They went back to the city and told everyone what they knew.

> *33 Then those who kept them fled; and they went away into the city and told everything, including what had happened to the demon-possessed men. 34 And behold, the whole city came out to meet Jesus. And when they saw Him, they begged Him to depart from their region. (Matthew 8:33–34)*

The scriptures clearly say that "the whole city came out to meet Jesus." Did that mean that every last person in the city—men, women, kids, and little babies—came out or is this also a type of descriptive language that is meant to convey the idea that lots and lots of people from the city came out?

As we read through the Bible, we need to get comfortable with what it is trying to tell us with each passage. Sometimes that will mean separating descriptive phenomenological language from historical narrative language.

Discussion Questions

1. Do you sometimes wish that the Bible had better descriptions and solutions to some modern-day problems, like a cure for cancer? If you were going to list your top three wishes for better descriptions, what would they be?

2. In the 1 Samuel verse about blacksmithing, do you suppose the Israelites were frustrated with God that He did not tell them how to do blacksmithing at least as well as the Philistines? Why do you suppose that God did not tell them?

3. Do you get frustrated by your lack of understanding of angelology? How does this lack of understanding affect your view of the rest of the Bible?

4. The expression of the sunrise is a classic example of phenomenological language. Why do you suppose that we still use language like that today, even though we know it is not scientifically correct?

5. What do you think about phrases in the Bible that say "everyone came out?" How do you know how to interpret them?

6. Based on this introductory study, how will you respond to a friend when he or she asks you, "Do you really take the Bible literally?"

In the Beginning, Without Form and Void

In the Beginning

The Bible begins with, "In the beginning God created the heavens and the earth" (Genesis 1:1). It is a rather different opening line for a serious book of literature. You may be more familiar with some other opening lines

It was the best of times, it was the worst of times… (*A Tale of Two Cities*, Charles Dickens, 1859)

It was a bright cold day in April, and the clocks were striking thirteen. (*Nineteen Eighty-Four*, George Orwell, 1949)

It was a dark and stormy night. (Snoopy)

Most of the time, the opening line of a book sets up the time period, the place, or the story that is about to unfold. In the Bible, it starts with God existing in the beginning. The story begins to unfold by talking about God. The first thing that we learn is that God existed before the beginning of everything else.

It is very difficult for us to comprehend something or someone preexisting the universe. For us, the universe is everything. It is all matter, energy, and time. It is very hard to grasp that God existed before there was matter, energy, and time. Can you imagine the beginning of time? If so, can you imagine the time before the beginning of time? This is quite a brain teaser.

The ancient Greek philosophers described it with "οὐδὲν ἐξ οὐδενός" or as we know it in Latin *ex nihilo nihil fit*. Out of nothing, nothing comes. The thinking behind this is that if there ever was "nothing" or "no thing," there cannot ever be any created matter, energy, or substance to create anything. After all, nothing is nothing! From nothing, nothing comes. Science is very clear on this.

Yet, the Bible begins with "In the beginning God created…." It does not tell us why God created, but the rest of Genesis Chapter 1 tells how God created the world, plants, animals, and humans for His pleasure, and when they were created, "it was good."

The Bible concludes the opening line with, "In the beginning God created the heavens and the earth." The heavens and the earth are a way of describing all that exists. The Biblical account continues with, "The earth was without form, and void, and darkness was on the face of the deep" (Genesis 1:2). Here is a really powerful way of describing the universe before it existed: "without form and void and darkness."

Take a few minutes to calm your breath, close your eyes, and empty your mind. Imagine that you are a great writer, and then imagine the words that you would use to describe the absolute nothingness that was before the universe came into being. All that we know does not exist; there is only void and darkness. Now imagine a self-existing Creator bringing all that is into existence purely for His great pleasure. How does this make you feel?

Discussion Questions

1. How do you think God brought everything into existence? Did He shout it, sing it, or just think it?

2. If you were an angel in heaven with God when He created the universe, what would have thrilled you the most, the creation of the stars, the oceans, the trees, or your favorite animal?

3. What created plant or animal makes you laugh? Perhaps the platypus?

4. What does the Creation tell you about God? What about His power, creative energy, or lovingkindness?

5. As you think about these things, how does your relationship with Him change?

Without Form and Void in Math and Science

The opening lines of Genesis are surprisingly chilling:

> *² In the beginning God created the heavens and the earth. ² The earth was without form, and void; and darkness was on the face of the deep. And the Spirit of God was hovering over the face of the waters. (Genesis 1:1–2)*

These opening lines start to explain what the universe was like before it was created. Yes, that is quite a brainteaser, describing something before it existed. Obviously, before it existed, it was no thing—nothing. But, how do you describe nothing?

The expression here is "without form, and void." The phrase "without form" is meant to capture the fact that it cannot be described. It has no form, nothing in common with the known physical world. It has no shape, no color, no size, no smell, no taste, and no form. The word "void" is meant to capture the idea of nothingness.

Humans have always had a difficult time with the void, the big Nothing. Even in mathematics, the very clever Romans had so much trouble with the idea of a void that they could not grasp the number zero. They were philosophically opposed to the idea of zero as a number. Every numeral needed to have a set of objects in the physical world that would correspond to the numeral. There was no such object that corresponded to the idea of zero. Hence, there is no Roman numeral for zero, but there are numerals for numbers like 9 and 10, IX, X.

The Romans and the Greeks struggled with the question, "How can not being be?"

Euclid, the great Greek mathematician, who is credited with the development of geometry, defined things like a straight line, a plane, a triangle, and a point. We all have a working definition of a point. For example, the period at the end of this sentence could be described as a point. However, in Euclid's geometry, a point is described as having no parts or magnitude. It is the punctuation that ends a sentence and at the same time has no dimensions, size, parts, or magnitude. In mathematics, we are still trying to figure out the correct mathematical definition of a point today.

We also struggle with the idea of the void today in astrophysics. As the science of the universe gets more and more complex, the idea of "empty space" recedes further and further into the background.

Space is no longer empty. It is filled with cosmic dust, light photons, neutrinos, gravitons, background radiation, and many other bits of mass and energy. The latest models have most of the universe filled with dark matter and dark energy.

We are not sure what dark matter is, but we think that we know what dark matter is not. It is not a cloud of matter without stars or planets, it is not antimatter, and it is not made up of black holes; yet, whatever it is, it interacts with gravity.

Dark energy is even more mysterious. So far, we know that we cannot detect it, measure it, or taste it. Yet, it seems to permeate all of the known universe in such massive quantities that it makes up about 70% of the entire universe. We believe that space is filled up but are still struggling to describe what it is filled up with.

It gets even more mysterious in some of the Big Bang theories, at the very beginning of time, the entire universe started to expand out from a singularity. In the very beginning, it was such a hot ball of energy that the current laws of physics did not apply at all. In fact, when it exploded into being (whatever that means), the light and energy were traveling much, much faster than the speed of light. A very, very short time after the Big Bang explosion, the entire universe was the size of a grapefruit. It makes one wonder, "What was outside this grapefruit-sized universe?" As the universe means all that is, this is quite a brain teaser.

It brings us back full circle to the idea of "without form and void." Perhaps this language at the beginning of the Bible is much more profound than we originally thought. This idea of "without form and void" merits much more thought and discussion.

Discussion Questions

1. Take a few moments to draw a picture of "without form and void". How did you do?

2. If you were to write a song about "without form and void," how would it go?

3. If you were given a school assignment to write a paragraph description of "without form and void," what would you write?

4. How would you help a Roman mathematician to understand the idea of zero?

5. If the entire universe was once the size of a very hot and energetic grapefruit, how would you describe what was outside the grapefruit?

6. What do all these thoughts tell us about God the Creator?

7. Based on what you see around you, does it make sense that all of the created world randomly exploded into being? How would you talk about this to a friend?

How Did the Universe Start?

What Is a Day and a Foundation?

One of the great controversies in faith and science is around the creation story in Genesis Chapter 1:

¹ In the beginning God created the heavens and the earth. ² The earth was without form, and void; and darkness was on the face of the deep. And the Spirit of God was hovering over the face of the waters.

³ Then God said, "Let there be light"; and there was light. ⁴ And God saw the light, that it was good; and God divided the light from the darkness. ⁵ God called the light Day, and the darkness He called Night. So the evening and the morning were the first day.

⁶ Then God said, "Let there be a firmament in the midst of the waters, and let it divide the waters from the waters." ⁷ Thus God made the firmament, and divided the waters which were under the firmament from the waters which were above the firmament; and it was so. ⁸ And God called the firmament Heaven. So the evening and the morning were the second day. (Genesis 1:1–8)

The Bible makes it clear that God preexisted the universe. He created all that is, out of a formless void. He started by creating light. He did this by speaking it into existence, "Let there be light." He then went on to create the firmament, the seas, the dry land, the grass, the trees, the sun, the moon, sea creatures, birds, land animals, and finally humans. Each of the creative days ends with the same phrase, for example, "So the evening and the morning were the second day." What exactly does this phrase mean?

The first key idea in these verses is the idea of separation, the light from the dark, or day from night. God calls the light good. It is good for many reasons, but one is that light is very important for all life. But He also calls each creative stage "day." What can that possibly mean?

The Hebrew word for day is *yom*. Unfortunately for us English speakers, the word *yom* seems to have lots of uses. In the beginning of these verses, *yom* is used for light. Then it is used for evening and morning, implying a day and night cycle.

14 Then God said, "Let there be lights in the firmament of the heavens to divide the day from the night; and let them be for signs and seasons, and for days and years; 15 and let them be for lights in the firmament of the heavens to give light on the earth"; and it was so. 16 Then God made two great lights: the greater light to rule the day, and the lesser light to rule the night. He made the stars also. 17 God set them in the firmament of the heavens to give light on the earth, 18 and to rule over the day and over the night, and to divide the light from the darkness. And God saw that it was good. 19 So the evening and the morning were the fourth day. (Genesis 1:14–19)

Then during the fourth creative day, the word *yom* is used repeatedly for daylight. The Hebrew word *yom* is very rich in meaning, and so sometimes its exact meaning can be a bit of a mystery.

For hundreds and hundreds of years, all of the great thinkers in the Church, St. Augustine, Francis of Assisi, John Wycliffe, Martin Luther, and John Calvin, to name just a few, all interpreted "evening and morning" to mean a full day cycle, what we would call 24 hours.

After the scientific revolutions in the 1700s and beyond, some Christian thinkers began to relook at the word *yom*. The way that we thought about the solar system and the entire universe began to change, and it forced us to reexamine how we read the opening section of Genesis. For example, science in the 1700s forced us to examine another Biblical concept— foundations.

Another tricky word in the Bible is "foundation." For example, in the Psalms, the Earth is described as having an unshakable foundation:

> *You who laid the foundations of the earth, So that it should not be moved forever… (Psalm 104:5)*

When Galileo and Copernicus turned the scientific world on its head with their idea that the Earth was not at the center of the solar system, but the Sun was, many people would not believe it. How could the Earth be orbiting around the Sun if it does not feel like it is moving? Everyone knew what it felt like to feel the wind on their face when they rode a horse. Why is that not happening if the Earth is moving around the Sun? Couple this confusion with the Biblical idea of the foundations of the Earth not being moved, and what is one to believe? All of the early Church fathers like Augustine, Aquinas, all the way up to John Calvin, and Martin Luther believed that the Earth was at the center of the solar system. After all, why wouldn't they if the Earth's foundation could not be moved?

Does the Bible say that the Earth is at the center of the solar system, or is it talking about the glory and power of God as the Creator? How do these ideas get reconciled?

Unfortunately, the debate continues. Surprisingly, God does not seem to be too focused on the mechanics of the creation story. He is much more concerned with the purpose of the creation and of mankind. Perhaps He is trying to tell us to focus back on "In the beginning God created…."

Discussion Questions

1. Why do you suppose God created all that is? Did He need to do it? Was He required to do it?

2. Could He do it on any timescale that He wanted to? How important is the creation timescale to God? If He was describing His timescale to the angels in heaven before the creation of the Earth, how would He describe it?

3. How would you convince Martin Luther or John Calvin that the Earth is not at the center of the solar system, nor is it at the center of our galaxy, the Milky Way?

4. How do these scientific debates relate to the character of God?

5. How do these debates affect your view of your purpose in the creation?

Spontaneous Generation

The early Greek philosophers, like Aristotle, thought deeply about a wide range of subjects. One particularly thorny issue was *where does life come from*? Without the aid of modern microscopes, it was easy to surmise that some organisms came directly out of the sand and mud. For example, Aristotle believed that scallops came directly out of the sand. The general thesis was that life comes from nonlife and that no causal agent was required. This seemed to explain a great deal of the world, especially some of the nastier creatures like fleas, mosquitos, and maggots. For most certainly maggots seemed to come directly out of decaying fish. We call this idea of organisms coming out of nothing on their own "spontaneous generation." This idea of spontaneous generation survived for thousands of years. Even the early Christian thinkers, such as St. Augustine, believed that spontaneous generation was described in some of the creation verses, such as, "Then God said, 'Let the waters abound with an abundance of living creatures....'" (Genesis 1:20a).

After all, the descriptive language seemed to say that creatures just came out the waters.

In the 1600s, the scientist Jan Baptist van Helmont did some interesting experiments with plants and mice. He planted a willow tree in a planter with a known amount of soil. He measured the growth of the willow tree for five years and compared its growth in mass to the loss in the mass of the soil. As the soil lost very little mass during this time, he concluded that the tree was spontaneously generating itself. He also concluded that mice could spontaneously generate from wheat scraps that were left in the garden shed. Aristotle's early ideas were very much entrenched in everyone's thinking.

In the mid-1800s, Louis Pasteur became very interested in the idea of spontaneous generation. He found that boiling meat could prevent the growth of mold and spores, and he eventually concluded his experiments with two significant ideas: one, there seem to be many small creatures (bacteria) living in decaying pieces of meat; and, two, boiling the meat could kill the small creatures. With this work, Pasteur did several things for science. First, he helped us to begin to understand microscopic life, such as bacteria. Second, he killed the idea of spontaneous generation, once and for all. From the mid-1800s to the mid-1900s, spontaneous generation was dead and buried.

Much to the surprise of many scientists, spontaneous generation came back to life along with the theory of the Big Bang. The Big Bang is often described as the universe *exploding into being*. It explodes out of nothing. Before the Big Bang, there is just a massless, dimensionless point (a singularity), and then *bang!* The universe comes into being. Unfortunately, science has said for over one hundred years that this cannot happen.

A related quandary for faith and science is the logical foundation of cause and effect. This logical principle states that every effect has an antecedent cause. If this is true, what is the cause of the Big Bang? On the other side of the coin, God does not need an antecedent cause as He is not an effect, but He is an eternal, self-existent Being.

These scientific ideas of spontaneous generation and cause and effect are quite a quandary for the scientific idea of the Big Bang. Where did the Big Bang come from? What started it? If there was a singularity with no mass or energy, how could the universe be formed from this starting point? The famous British physicist, Stephen Hawking, is purported to say that before the Big Bang, there was absolutely nothing. This is quite an interesting scientific and philosophical quandary. Is spontaneous generation back on the table?

Perhaps "In the beginning God..." is beginning to make scientific sense.

Discussion Questions

1. Do things exist even though we cannot see them? How do you know?

2. Do you think that scientists have a hard or easy time changing their theories? Why?

3. How would you engage a Big Bang scientist on the idea of "exploding into being"?

4. Is Genesis Chapter 1 relevant to the Big Bang theory? If so, what are the implications?

The Knowledge of the Ancients

Did the Ancients Know Science?

We often declare today that the ancients did not know much about science. Nothing could be further from the truth! Our understanding of the ancients is clouded by our view of the Dark Ages. During the Dark Ages, much of what the Greeks had known was lost.

In the 1400s and early 1500s, most people thought that the Earth was flat. This is why the journey of Magellan around the world in 1522 was so significant. He resurrected some very early knowledge of the Greeks.

Not only did the Greeks know that the Earth was round, but they actually calculated the circumference of the Earth. In 230 BC, Eratosthenes made a very interesting observation. At noon on the summer solstices, the sun was directly overhead of a specific well in the city of Syene. This was quite a sight, as everyone in the town would flock to look down the well and see a perfect image of the sun at the bottom of the well, just one day every year.

One year on the summer solstice, Eratosthenes was in a different city, Alexandria. He expected to join in the celebration in that city, at their central well. However, instead of finding a central well with no shadow, he found that every building, well, and tower had a shadow. He measured some of the shadows and found them all to be at 7.2° and not 0°. Eratosthenes thought about this for a while and decided that the only way that this could happen is if Alexandria is "falling away" from Syene. In other words, the Earth is curved and not flat.

Eratosthenes then hired a professional walker to walk from Alexandria to Syene. The walker measured the distance between the two cities to be 490 miles. Eratosthenes then calculated the radius of the Earth to be 3,900 miles. This is only 2% off of the modern value for the radius of the Earth of 3,960 miles. Amazing!

As you can see, Jesus and his disciples grew up in a time of great scientific knowledge and understanding. That is one of the reasons that the narrative of Jesus walking on the water is so significant.

[22] Immediately Jesus made His disciples get into the boat and go before Him to the other side, while He sent the multitudes away. [23] And when He had sent the multitudes away, He went up on the mountain by Himself to pray. Now when evening came, He was alone there. [24] But the boat was now in the middle of the sea, tossed by the waves, for the wind was contrary.

[25] Now in the fourth watch of the night Jesus went to them, walking on the sea. [26] And when the disciples saw Him walking on the sea, they were troubled, saying, "It is a ghost!" And they cried out for fear.

[27] But immediately Jesus spoke to them, saying, "Be of good cheer! It is I; do not be afraid."

[33] Then those who were in the boat came and worshiped Him, saying, "Truly You are the Son of God." (Matthew 14:22–27, 33)

The disciples in the boat were experienced fishermen. Until Jesus showed up in their lives, that was all they knew. They knew the Sea of Galilee like the back of their hands. They knew the properties of buoyance and water density. They knew what floated and what did not. They knew that you could swim in the Sea of Galilee but you could not walk on top of it.

So, when they saw Jesus walking on top of the water, their first thought was that He was a ghost, because what else could it be? For we know from Occam's razor that this simplest explanation is often the best. However, in this case, they were surprised that it was a man, Jesus Himself.

Once they recovered from their fear, they recognized Jesus as the Son of God. Does this discussion help you to see that the miracles in the Bible might make more sense?

Discussion Questions

1. Why do you think that most people today believe that the ancients did not know scientific principles and were basically ignorant?

2. Could you calculate the size of the Earth with just a stick and a protractor? If not, who would you get to help you?

3. If you were in the boat with the disciples, what would you have said when you saw Jesus walking on the water, and why?

4. If your neighbors saw Jesus walking on the water, would it convince them that God is real? Why or why not?

The Ancient's View of Death and Miracles

We often wonder, what did the ancients know about death and miracles? The everyday individual in Jesus' time knew so much more about death than we do today. Therefore, they would definitely know a resurrection miracle if they saw one.

While children under one year old do die today, it is not very common. In ancient Roman times, one-quarter to one-third of the children did not live past their first year. Almost all children grew up watching a younger sibling die. Almost all children attended a funeral every year for some young person either in their family or in their village. Children grew up knowing about death.

If they were lucky enough to make it past their first year, they might live to be twenty-five years old, as that was the average life expectance of someone in ancient Rome. While some elders in each village made it into their fifties or sixties, this was rare. Everyone saw death as a common part of everyday life. Everyone participated in preparing a body for burial and designing a funeral service.

This is why the encounter between a particular Jewish religious ruler and Jesus was very unusual. The religious ruler knew that his daughter was dead. He probably watched her die. As other family members were preparing the young girl's body for burial, he rushed out to find this new traveling rabbi, Jesus. When he found Jesus, he told Jesus to come and lay His hands on his daughter so that she would live again.

[18] While He spoke these things to them, behold, a ruler came and worshiped Him, saying, "My daughter has just died, but come and lay Your hand on her and she will live." [19] So Jesus arose and followed him, and so did His disciples.

[23] When Jesus came into the ruler's house, and saw the flute players and the noisy crowd wailing, [24] He said to them, "Make room, for the girl is not dead, but sleeping." And they ridiculed Him. [25] But when the crowd was put outside, He went in and took her by the hand, and the girl arose. [26] And the report of this went out into all that land. (Matthew 9:18–19, 23–26)

When Jesus got to this man's house, the funeral procession was in full swing. The professional mourners of the day, the flute players, and the noisy crowd were in the middle of a full performance for honoring the departed girl. Jesus asked for them to make room because the girl was not dead, as He was going to bring her back to life. The mourners laughed at Jesus. They knew death. They knew a dead body. They knew the feel of rigor mortis, the smell; they knew death as a part of everyday life.

Jesus put them outside of the room. He probably spoke to the girl and asked her to take His hand.

He then reached out and took her hand, and she squeezed His fingers. Her heart started beating, and she started breathing again. After a few moments, she probably opened her eyes and looked at the face of Jesus. They probably smiled together, and then she swung her feet off of the bed and got up.

The last line of this story is the most important: "The report of this went out into all that land." Everyone there knew that a miracle happened. Jesus used these miracles as a sign to point to His work with His Father. He came to Earth to do some remarkable things. Everyone there that day knew without a shadow of a doubt that a miracle happened.

Discussion Questions

1. Have you been around death? Would you have been like the Jewish religious ruler and gone out on a limb and publicly asked for a miracle?

2. Why doesn't God do miracles like this every time we ask?

3. Everyone, the professional mourners, the friends of the family, and most importantly the father, knew that Jesus had done a great miracle, the greatest miracle. He brought someone back to life. What does this mean to us today?

4. If you and your neighbors saw a miracle like this, what would everyone think?

5. What does it mean for us today that Jesus did real miracles while He was on Earth?

Made in God's Image

In God's Image or Wholly Other?

God declares that we are made in His image:

> *26 Then God said, "Let Us make man in Our image, according to Our likeness; let them have dominion over the fish of the sea, over the birds of the air, and over the cattle, over all the earth and over every creeping thing that creeps on the earth."*

> *27 So God created man in His own image; in the image of God He created him; male and female He created them. 28 Then God blessed them, and God said to them, "Be fruitful and multiply; fill the earth and subdue it; have dominion over the fish of the sea, over the birds of the air, and*

over every living thing that moves on the earth."
(Genesis 1:26–28)

What does it mean to be made in the image of someone else or to have their likeness? When it comes to humans, we can often see how a baby looks like one or both of his or her parents. We often see the eyes of one parent and the ears of the other on the face of a baby. But, what does it mean to be made in God's image?

Thinkers throughout the ages have quickly discarded the idea that we have eyes or ears like our Creator. For one, we are all too different. For another, He must be so much bigger than us that it does not make sense that He has a face, arms, and hands as we do.

In general, the great thinkers have come to believe that this means that we are created with intelligence. We are moral agents. We have a conscience. We all understand the concept of fairness. We all have a will, and we can execute our wills and desires. We have hearts filled with emotions and passion. We understand what love is, even though we have trouble defining it. We have the ability to create art and beauty. We all know how to laugh no matter what part of the world we live in. All of these characteristics are attributes of God described throughout various parts of the Bible.

However, various theologians have struggled deeply with the idea of being made in God's image.

One in particular, Karl Barth, wrote in the early 1900s that God must be "wholly other." Barth argued that God must be so much more intelligent, worthy, holy, loving, and so on than us and that He must be completely different from us. Some have made the argument that God is so far beyond us that we cannot comprehend Him. They say that you cannot compare a Deity to humans; He is much too big compared to us. The comparison is more like a human compared to an amoeba. Sure, an amoeba has locomotion and perhaps has a will, but the intellectual gap between humans and amoebas is so great that there is no way in which a human could communicate with an amoeba, nor is there a way in which an amoeba could reach up to a human.

Karl Barth does a great job of expanding on the greatness of God and His immensity; however, he misses the point that God over and over again tells His people in the Bible that He loves them deeply. Therefore, there must be some connection points between the Creator and the creatures. Because of His greatness, He must be the One to connect with the human. We are too small and unworthy to connect with Him on our own. Therefore, He has reached out over hundreds of years with special prophets, spokesmen, and finally His own Son. This is one of the reasons why the incarnation is such an important concept in the Christian Church.

Modern scientists are beginning to understand just how big the entire universe is. We get a small glimpse of this when we look at all of the stars on a very clear night. If God the Creator made all of this, how could we possibly reach out to comprehend Him? A question for the scientist is then, "Just because He must be so much bigger than us, does that mean that He does not exist?"

Discussion Questions

1. If you were given a research grant to communicate with amoeba, how would you begin?

2. If you were an angel in heaven and you were given the task to describe God the Creator to humans, what method would you emphasize? Pictures, songs, words, stories, or some other method?

3. Must the Creator be able to speak and understand all languages? If so, how do you think we will communicate with God and each other in heaven? One universal language, our own language, telepathically, or some other method?

4. How does the vastness of the universe make you feel?

How Do We Cover Our Shame?

Almost everyone has heard about the fig leaves that Adam and Eve used to cover themselves. The story can be found in Genesis 3:

> *⁶ So when the woman saw that the tree was good for food, that it was [pleasant to the eyes, and a tree desirable to make one wise, she took of its fruit and ate. She also gave to her husband with her, and he ate. ⁷ Then the eyes of both of them were opened, and they knew that they were naked; and they sewed fig leaves together and made themselves coverings. (Genesis 3:6–7)*

Eve disobeyed a direct command from God not to eat from that one tree. There were lots of other trees to eat from, but as we are ought to do, Adam and Eve thought that their freedoms were being impinged on by not being allowed to do everything that they wanted. They represented us as usurpers. We all rebel against restrictions to our freedom, and often we will go out of our way to break any rule that is limiting our lives.

In this case, once they disobeyed God's direct command, they realized their true, rebellious nature and they were ashamed. The word used here is *naked*, which in this context means *totally exposed.* To hide their guilt and shame, they made fig leaf garments to try to cover themselves.

Personal guilt, *I know that I have done something wrong,* and personal shame, *I know that I am a bad person*, are very hard to deal with. Modern psychology has been trying to help us deal with our guilt and shame for a long time, with mixed results.

Sigmund Freud (1856–1939) is known to be the father of psychoanalysis. He thought that our problems of guilt and shame came from deep-seated relational problems with our parents. He proposed that there was also an internal battle between our id, which is focused on our personal pleasure, our ego, which helps us deal with reality, and our superego, which might be thought of as our conscience. While these are helpful insights into some of Freud's ideas, they do not deal with the root problem of our guilt and shame. He did not offer any way to remove our guilt and shame. We all found that our guilt and shame do not go away by just talking about the problem.

BF Skinner (1904–1990) came about fifty years later. He taught that free will was an illusion. Our actions are determined by positive or negative reinforcement. While this was a good philosophy for helping to modify behavior, like in children, he did not help us once we had done something wrong. There is no way to behaviorally modify guilt and shame away. Again, while these were helpful insights on how we can modify the behavior of others, Skinner did not help us deal with the problem of our own guilt and shame.

Jean Piaget (1896–1980) was a contemporary of Skinner. Piaget was all about education. He believed that education was capable of saving our societies from total collapse. He thought that we could educate proper behavior. Again, while these were helpful insights on how to modify behavior, he did not help us deal with our mistakes. Often, we know what wrong is, but we do it anyway. We have a strong sense of oughtness, what we ought to do in any given situation, yet we cannot always make ourselves do what we ought to do. Piaget's ideas did not help us deal with our guilt and shame.

The story in Genesis continues with God punishing Adam, Eve, and the serpent for their transgressions. After declaring the punishment, He comes alongside Adam and Eve and gives them a way to deal with their guilt and shame. First, he covers them.

Also for Adam and his wife the Lord *God made tunics of skin, and clothed them. (Genesis 3:21)*

He allows them to cover themselves and then control how they expose their innermost selves to others as they saw fit. We see this in our own lives today. With acquaintances, we allow them to see the high-level, basic parts of our lives. With very close friends, we allow them to see more of our inner lives, even the parts that expose some of our weaknesses and darkness. In our most intimate relationships, we can expose more of our inner selves, but even in these relationships, we sometimes hold things back. However, God allows us to share everything about ourselves with Him. If we confess our wrongdoings to Him and ask for forgiveness, He will take our guilt and shame upon Himself and remove it from us. He is able to wash us clean and make us white as snow. God gives us a way to deal with our guilt and shame, He offers to take away from us.

...Though your sins are like scarlet, they shall be as white as snow; though they are red like crimson, they shall be as wool. (Isaiah 1:18)

God is the only one who can take our guilt and shame and remove it from us "as far as the east is from the west" (Psalm 103:12). Science has been struggling with the problem of guilt and shame for a very long time, with very poor success.

Discussion Questions

1. Have you seen guilt and shame destroy a friend or acquaintance? How would you describe the impact of guilt and shame on their lives?

2. How would you describe a common method used in society today to cover our guilt and shame? Why does this not work very well?

3. Why does God always tell us that He must help us deal with our guilt and shame? How do verses like Isaiah 1:18 "white as snow" make you feel?

4. What would the world be like if we thought that the weight of our guilt and shame might never be lifted?

More About God's Image

Are We Unique?

When people hear about men and women being made in God's image, they often ask, "well, what about __________ (fill in your favorite animal)?"

We often talk about special properties that we have—intelligence, passion, creativity, love for art, love for others, our ability to exert our will, and unfortunately our ability to feel shame and guilt.

We often talk about animals that exhibit intelligence. We have seen how smart and caring some animals are like dolphins and elephants. We have seen animals expressing love and concern, especially our dogs and cats. We have seen tool-making in animals such as clever crows. So, what makes us so special? The Bible would describe it as a matter of degree.

In the Book of Isaiah, God describes Himself compared to us like this:

> *8 "For My thoughts are not your thoughts,*
> *Nor are your ways My ways," says the* LORD.
> *9 "For as the heavens are higher than the earth,*
> *So are My ways higher than your ways,*
> *And My thoughts than your thoughts.*
> *(Isaiah 55:8–9)*

God is telling us that we have thoughts—important thoughts. We exercise our wills. It is just that His thoughts and His ways are so beyond us; it is like the separation between heaven, where He lives, and earth, where we live.

In the Book of Job, God gives several other clear examples:

> *4 "Where were you when I laid the foundations*
> *of the earth?*
> *Tell Me, if you have understanding.*
> *5 Who determined its measurements?*
> *Surely you know!*
> *Or who stretched the [b]line upon it?*
> *6 To what were its foundations fastened?*
> *Or who laid its cornerstone,*
> *7 When the morning stars sang together,*
> *And all the sons of God shouted for joy?*
> *(Job 38:4–7)*

God makes it clear that He made the universe and the earth with great care. He laid the foundations. He measured it to make sure it was right. He created the stars and galaxies so that they may sing to His glory. Yes, we can create things, but can we create an entire universe? Can we bring a star into being and make it sing with joy?

Can you bind the cluster of the Pleiades, Or loose the belt of Orion? (Job 38:31)

A little later on in the discourse, He challenges Job to undo (loosen) the belt of Orion. Orion is a huge wintertime constellation that dominates the night sky. It is made of many different stars. The belt is made of three stars that appear to be in a straight line. God tells us all something like, *If you think you are so great, make another Orion in the sky, or undo his belt.*

God uses these descriptions to make us understand how vastly different He is from us. In the same way, we have things in common with the animal kingdom, but we are vastly different from them.

When the animals look at the stars at night, do they contemplate the constellations and ponder Orion's belt? Do they ponder the foundation of the earth? Do they ponder the size of the universe or how long it has existed? Do they see the stars singing together? Do they see beauty in a spectacular sunrise? Do they contemplate what it will be like to live on the planet Mars?

These are small pieces of what it means to be made in God's image.

So, enjoy your relationships with your animal friends, but more importantly, consider what it means that all men and women are made in God's image, those that you love, those you do not like, and those whom you hate. They are all made in God's image.

Discussion Questions

1. Imagine that you see a friend out walking their dog. How would you describe to them how uniquely both of you are made in the image of God, so much more so than their dog?

2. How would you describe how much more is God's love for them than their love for their dog?

3. What do you think about the idea that God expects you to love other people much more than your animal friends? Even those people that you do not like?

4. Can you think of people you know (that you don't like) that God might want you to reflect His love to? How could you do that, practically speaking? How might this impact them? How might this impact you?

What Is a Soul?

In Genesis Chapter 2, the creation of Adam is described using this line: "And the LORD God formed man of the dust of the ground, and breathed into his nostrils the breath of life, and man became a living being" (Genesis 2:7). Everyone wonders what the "breath of life" means. It is a bit difficult to understand because it is an old Hebrew expression and there are several aspects of this expression.

First, we see that God Himself breathed into the man so that he might become a living being. God could have just had the four winds blow into the man, or He could have given him a sharp spanking. However, God did something much more personal—He breathed into his nostrils. This is an expansion of what it means to be made into the image of God (Genesis 1:27). God did something special to the man and by extension to all of us by giving us the breath of life.

Another understanding of the verse is to see the idea of body and soul. We are not just physical creatures, nor are we just intellectual or spiritual creatures. The idea of body and soul was a big problem for Greek philosophers. According to Plato, the soul gave us reason, spirit, and appetites. The soul was the life driver for us all. At times, Plato abhorred the physical body as it was often in conflict with the soul.

These ideas of Plato are still very much alive today, in our modern world views. At times we hate our bodies. They are not what we want. They are too big, too small; too fat, too thin; they are too weak, too inflexible; their desires are too strong, and they often lead us astray.

For example, our spirit, mind, or soul keeps telling us to stay away from temptation, like the next drink or drug, but our body is too weak and we cave to the temptation. Like in Plato's time, we live with our spirit in conflict with our bodies.

The view in Genesis is quite different in that there is complete unity between body and spirit. God made both, and He gave us both. Sometimes, God's creative activity is described as a potter forming a vessel out of clay. The Potter meticulously forms the vessel for a specific purpose. Not all vessels are the same; they do not look the same, but they each have their own specific purpose. When God created us, He created us to be engaged in purposeful activities, and through these, we would find our meaning. The spirit needs the body, and the body needs the spirit.

Then Darwin came along with his evolutionary theory. In his theory, we all evolved from the primordial goop. Today we see that we not only share a lot of DNA with the apes, but we also share DNA with fruit flies. The explanation is that as we all have a great deal of commonality; therefore, we must all be the same.

There are two major weaknesses to this theory. The first is that just because there is a great deal of commonality that does not necessarily mean that we are all the same. After all, we are all carbon-based organisms, so it only makes sense that we would have a great deal of commonality. We would expect to have less commonality with nitrogen-based organisms.

The second weakness is around the idea of body and soul, or body and spirit. We cannot wrap our heads around the idea of bacteria or viruses having a soul. They do not seem to have a complex enough body to house a soul. So, that brings up a host of questions:

- Which organisms have a soul?
- Where did this soul come from?
- Did it just randomly happen one day? If so, how does a random event like this have any meaning?
- How do you randomly make a soul?
- Plato had the idea that the soul outlived the body. What would Darwin think about this?

The idea of the soul and the conscience was very troubling for Darwin. He could not figure out how the conscience could randomly evolve, as the conscience would sometimes drive people to sacrifice themselves for someone else, which went against his idea of the all-powerful drive for self-preservation. Darwin had no answers to the perplexing questions above, and they still stump many scientists today.

It seems that the Judeo-Christian idea of the breath of life better answers many of these questions and most clearly answers the following questions:

- Why does life matter?
- How do you put together the ideas of body and soul?
- How can you bring better unity between your body and soul?

Discussion Questions

1. If you were given the debate question, "In Darwin's evolutionary theory, when did the soul come into existence?", describe your approach to answering this question.

2. It has been said that humans have a great deal of DNA in common with gorillas. How would you use this information to explain that we are uniquely made in God's image?

3. Do you see the conscience as a good thing for humans? If so, why?

4. What excites you about the idea that the soul outlives the body?

Rise from the Dead?

A significant keystone pillar of Christianity is that Jesus rose from the dead. This is awfully hard to believe as it is something that just does not occur in everyday life.

The counterclaims to the stories from Jesus' followers of Him rising from the dead follow a few different paths.

First is that Jesus did not really die. He just swooned in the tomb for three days, and during that time His body healed itself and He fooled everyone. Medical science has debunked this idea based on the nature of His death. He was killed by crucifixion, which was the most horrific death for criminals that the Romans could come up with. Crucifixion was a slow and painful death, generally coming from suffocation because the criminal could no longer push his body up to take a breath. In Jesus' case, He was flogged with a cat-o'-nine-tails so that he was bleeding severely from wounds on His back. Medical science agrees that no one could recover from flogging and crucifixion in three days with no food, water, or medical attention.

Another idea is that the followers stole His body and then agreed to just make up a story about His resurrection. This does not hold psychological weight in that ten of His original followers were tortured horribly for their faith and not one of them cracked under the torture. Psychologists agree that at least one of them, if not all of them, would have cracked under the pressure if they knew that the resurrection story was fake. They would have had no reason to keep propagating the story of His resurrection. Except for face-saving, they had nothing to gain from His resurrection stories. If they knew that the resurrection story was false, they would have just gone back to their previous employment. For example, Peter was a fisherman. If he could abandon the story of Jesus' resurrection, he would get his wife, his family, and his job and get his old life back. However, he held fast to the fact that Jesus rose from the dead. He saw the empty tomb, and he saw the resurrected Jesus, multiple times. So, he stuck to the story, even when tortured to death.

Perhaps the most surprising attempt to explain away Jesus' resurrection was from the religious community. The religious leaders, the chief priest, and the elders came up with a plan to bribe the Roman soldiers who were guarding the tomb where Jesus was buried. The soldiers were to tell anyone who asked

His disciples came at night and stole Him away while they slept. (Matthew 28:11–15)

It is incredible to imagine this storyline. These Roman soldiers were some of the best of the best. They would never fall asleep while at their post. Most certainly, they would not all fall asleep at the same time while at their posts. This would be like all of the Secret Service agents guarding a very important person, like a president or vice president, falling asleep on the job. Can you imagine the newspaper headlines the next day? "The President was kidnapped while the Secret Service agents slept." These agents could never face life again. They could not face their fellow agents, their families, or anyone in the community. It would have been the same for the Roman soldiers. Clearly, this story does not hold water.

The Christian faith is an evidence-based faith. This can be seen in Thomas' encounter with the resurrected Jesus.

[24] Now Thomas, called the Twin, one of the twelve, was not with them when Jesus came. [25] The other disciples therefore said to him, "We have seen the Lord."

So he said to them, "Unless I see in His hands the print of the nails, and put my finger into the print of the nails, and put my hand into His side, I will not believe."

²⁶ And after eight days His disciples were again inside, and Thomas with them. Jesus came, the doors being shut, and stood in the midst, and said, "Peace to you!" ²⁷ Then He said to Thomas, "Reach your finger here, and look at My hands; and reach your hand here, and put it into My side. Do not be unbelieving, but believing."

²⁸ And Thomas answered and said to Him, "My Lord and my God!" (John 20:24–28)

Thomas based his faith on real scientific evidence. He demanded to see the resurrected Jesus, and he saw and touched. He had his evidence!

Using Occam's razor, we would have to agree that the simplest explanation for Jesus' resurrection is best.

Discussion Questions

1. Are there other explanations for Jesus' resurrection? How do they stack up to a scientific inquiry?

2. What does it mean if this resurrection story is just a hoax?

3. The most logical explanation is that Jesus actually did rise from the dead. If this is true, what does it mean for your life?

Other Books by TS Taylor

Life-Changing Devotionals

The Love and Mercy of God as Seen in Jonah,
Job, and Joseph

Flight to Freedom, Laws to Live By, How to Worship

Exodus Devotionals

High and Lifted Up – Is God Still
Engaged in His World?

Isaiah Devotionals

Walk with Jesus and His Followers

Matthew Devotional

Life Applications from Romans

Romans Devotional